IVETTE BROWN

B-Wellness

365 SELF CARE

Journal

ANATOMY OF LIFESTYLE
HEALTH PLANNER

*A Mind-Body approach to
achieving Holistic Health*

Acknowledgements:

This book would not have been possible without my partner in life and best friend who pushes me to be my best everyday. I humbly thank you and love you for eternity! A special thanks to my mother, family members and extended family for their continued support. I appreciate you all.

TABLE OF CONTENTS

12 months January-December

4-part planner/calendar/book

Designed to teach mindful wellness practices for daily use

It includes Nutrition, Recipes, Exercise Routines, Monthly cooking themes, challenges and self care recommendations.

We focus on the "WE" in wellness because we recognize our connection to communities worldwide. Use this self care system to evaluate your own health & wellness.

This book is appropriate for individual's age's 5-& up who are seeking a holistic approach to obtain optimal health. Recommend this to families as well. We are teaching communities to Live Mindful/Eat Mindful/Being Mindful of everyday choices and actions.

Today starts 12 Months of Wellness

Thank you for making the choice to improve your wellness! Today you will start your 12 months of B-Wellness365 self care system, which means everyday for the next 12 months is a new day to reach your wellness goals.

B-Wellness365 is a 12-Month Mindful health planner and journal designed to help families, individuals or anyone with goals to change and improve their health and well being.

This Year Mindful health planner will help you in every season and/ has 12 activities themed topics around health, nutrition, physical fitness, growth mindset, kindness, self-love, gratitude and monthly challenges.

Before starting each topic monthly make a commitment to complete the chapters without skipping any (if possible)

Remember that you have the right to be well for the rest of your life!

The purpose of this book is for as many people as possible to experience the benefits of overall wellness and fitness including individuals, youth and families in a structured way, with me "Brownie Wellness" as your accountability partner guiding you along your journey!

Each month is filled with a colored theme to engage together and practice doing your best being a healthy family or a healthy individual. Experience the true synergy between Mind, Body and Health with this journal planner.

We have put together a wellness offering list with information about our classes, workshops and programs to help you on this journey. We have designed opportunities for you to continue your wellness commitment program with on-line and in-person support. I am so happy that you've chosen to take this journey to improve your quality of life!

Your future self thanks you and I am honored to be on this wellness journey with you.

Commitment Contract

<u>How do you plan to achieve your goals this year?</u>

This 12 Step Mindful Wellness Program is designed to help you achieve your own state of wellness. This health planner also offers you a blueprint for achieving success with our 12 Monthly Themes, Tips, Holidays, Challenges, and Holidays/Events to keep you on track every month.

This book is appropriate for individual's age's 5-& up who are seeking a holistic approach to obtain optimal health..

I recommend this book to families to implement. We focus on the "WE" in wellness because we recognize our connection to communities worldwide. B-Wellness365 journal is teaching communities to Live Mindful/Eat Mindful/ by Being Mindful of our everyday choices and actions. Use this self care system to evaluate your own health & wellness

1.

2.

3.

4.

5.

6.

7.

8.

9.

10.

11.

12.

Sign and Date _____

I am committing to complete this journey and will NOT give up!

Outline of Chapters

The book is broken down into the following monthly categories:

Color:
Muscle:
Food:
Exercise:
Recommendation/Tip:
Holiday
Goal:

Part1: chapters 1-3

1. Attitudes and Values of Health

2. Behavioral Management

3. Self Care or Welfare

Part 2: chapters 4-6

4. Mindless vs Mindful behavior

5. Stress overload

6. Meditation Minutes (M&M time) & rest

Part 3: chapters 7-8

7. Choosing wellness over wackiness

8. Just Breathe

Part 4: chapters 9-12

Preface:

As the New Year approaches, some people make resolutions that are incomplete by the end of January. This book will help guide you every month. This flexible planner grows with you. Keep it simple or challenge yourself. It's up to you!

Let's work together to help make this year your best year ever by using this Health Planner Journal to be your accountability partner for the next 12 months. Use this 12 Month Meditation and Self-Care Curriculum Guide on your health journey to achieve your everyday wellness goals. Healing is a journey and it requires intelligent and guided action, not guessing. It requires listening to your body, then taking that feedback to make adjustments and work toward improvements.

Life can be very stressful and people are in search of positive ways to deal with stress. I realize mindfulness, meditation, mental health and self -care is a life long journey and believe that mental, physical and spiritual health is key to living a successful life.

Practice

Self-mastery
Self care
Self defense
Self-reflection
Self-motivation
Self help

Let us help you develop your health plan this year

Definitions:

Holistic, Wellness, Mindfulness, Self Care

PART 1

Numerous studies show a positive association between physical activity and public health, including improved physical health, mental health, and social stability (Cohen, Boniface, and Watkins, 2014; Mindell et al., 2014).

CHAPTER 1:

Attitudes and Values of Health

When we choose our attitude towards our health, things tend to shift.

You learn to look at the better side of things, and evaluate things.

You also develop:

- Optimistic views
- Focus on the positive
- See things differently
- Change 1 thing at a time

You begin to understand that there are no such things as quick fixes, and you begin to feel Issues of concern, and need to find a Safe space to open up. Once you feel:

- Stability
- Support
- Regulation

You will be able to make a transformation that will last!

What are some of your our attitude towards your own health?

Share your thoughts......

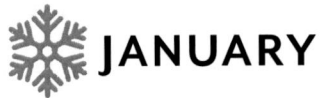 JANUARY

January is New Years & MLK birthday, & national soup month

This month's theme is: Jump into January! This is a new year to jumpstart your goals! Vision boards are a great way to create a storyboard for your Goal Setting to remind you of your goals visually.

This month's theme color is White and the symbol is Snow Flake.

Try eating white color foods such as Cauliflower, Lychee, or White onions.

January's muscle of the month is the Lattisimus Dorsi muscle, which are located in the back. Try performing a Bridge, Pull Ups, Deadlifts, or Seated Rows to target the back muscles.

January is about aiming high to achieve new results. Take one step at time and set SMART goals that are specific, measurable, achievable, realistic and timely! When you create your Vision Board to visualize this goal and start the New Year off with accountability and are inspired.

Happy New Year and Happy Birthday to everyone celebrating a birthday this month!

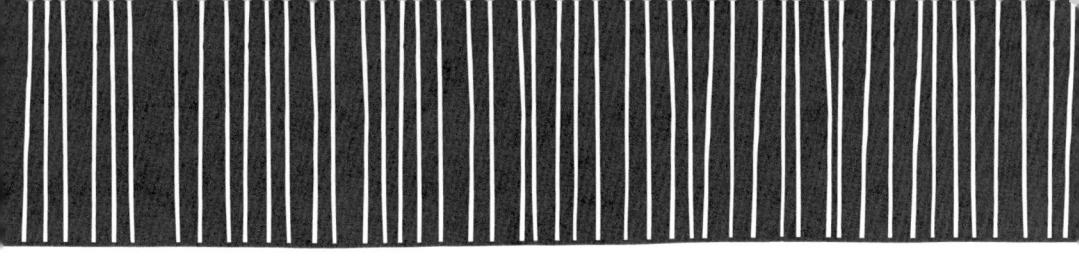

CHAPTER 2:

Behavioral Management

B-Wellness daily commitment wellness mantra

I am mindful of my wellness and I plan today to be well by doing the following things.

1. _____
2. _____
3. _____

Fill in the blank...

My wellness is:_____

My own responsibility: _____
My own right: _____
My own journey: _____

I empower _____

I educate _____

I help _____

I heal _____

I care _____

I am B-Wellness365 your name: _____

For this month, my goal is to _____

Love and Light *Ivette Brown*

Love & Light Questionnaire

Assess your answers

Do you make a difference in the lives of others? If so, How?

_____

_____

_____

How do you practice self care?

_____

_____

_____

Do you live your life with generosity?

_____

_____

_____

_____

Do you help causes that help people?

_____

_____

_____

Have you given, time talent or resources is a form of generosity?

_____

_____

_____

Do you see the value in yourself and others?

_____

_____

_____

How important is Wellness to you?

_____

_____

_____

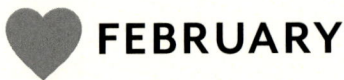 # FEBRUARY

February is National Heart month and dental health month.

It is also Black history month, & Chinese New Year, Ground hog day, Valentine's, Presidents' Day & Washington's Birthday month & Super Bowl

This month's theme is Fearless February

Our goal this month is to develop A Heart healthy lifestyle.

February's muscle of the month is the Aorta, also known as the heart muscle. Make sure to do exercises to strengthen your heart by doing cardiovascular activities such as cycling, jogging, walking or an aerobic class. Also try to eat foods like red bell pepper, cherries, strawberries, pomegranate, and beets for calcium and vitamin C this month.

February's color is: Red and its symbol is a Red Heart.

Happy Birthday to everyone celebrating a birthday this month!

February Goal sheet

I am mindful of my wellness and I plan today to be well today by doing the following things:

1. _____
2. _____
3. _____

Fill in the blank...

My wellness is:_____

My own responsibility: _____
My own right: _____
My own journey: _____

I empower _____

I educate _____

I help _____

I heal _____

I care _____

I am B-Wellness365 your name: _____

For this month, my goal is to _____

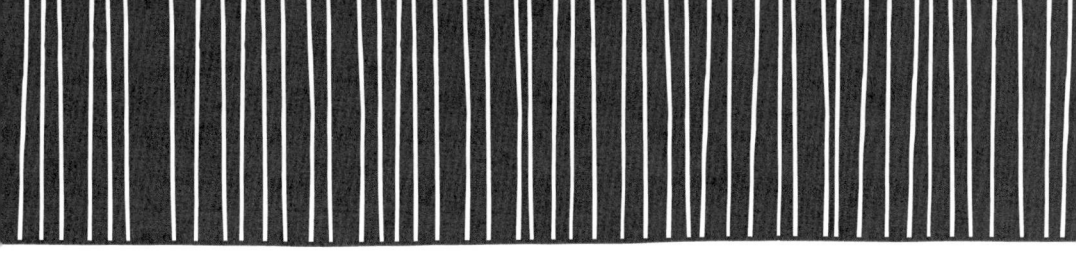

CHAPTER 3:

Self Care or Welfare

Self Care is defined as: the practice of taking action to preserve or improve one's own health.

When you decide self-care, you make a conscious decision to improve your quality of life. Self care focuses on knowledge of self and decision-making which recognizes that change is necessary rather than choosing to ignore the signs and symptoms that may occur.

Welfare is defined as the health, happiness and fortunes of a person or particular group. It is also defined as a means of financial support given to people in need.

Choosing self-care is the best decision that one can make because it empowers individuals to be proactive and can change the trajectory of their life. My suggestion is to choose a holistic approach to address the entire person including physical, mental and emotional health.

Holistic

Holistic refers to a whole or whole body; taking into consideration the whole body or person. According to Webster's dictionary Holistic means, of or relating to Holism. Emphasizing the importance of the whole and the interdependence of its parts.

Holistic approaches to health consider the mind, body and spirit.

Now ask yourself, have you been practicing self care or welfare? Share your thoughts.

 # MARCH

This month's theme is Mindfulness March. For this month of March Let's Go green and learn to Let Go

March's holidays/events are St. Patrick's Day & Easter, & Dr. Seuss birthday 3/2, & Women's history month and March madness month of basketball.

This month's theme symbol is a shamrock and the color is Green.

My recommendation is to try eating green foods like Kale, Collards, or green bell peppers.

The muscle of the month is Deltoids, which are located in the shoulder.

Try Lateral Raises, and Front Raises to strengthen the shoulder muscles.

Happy Birthday to everyone celebrating a birthday this month!

PART 2

March Goal Sheet

I am mindful of my wellness and I plan today to be well today by doing the following things:

1.

2.

3.

Fill in the blank...

My wellness is:_____

My own responsibility: _____
My own right: _____
My own journey: _____

I empower _____

I educate _____

I help _____

I heal _____

I care _____

I am B-Wellness365 your name: _____

For this month, my goal is to _____

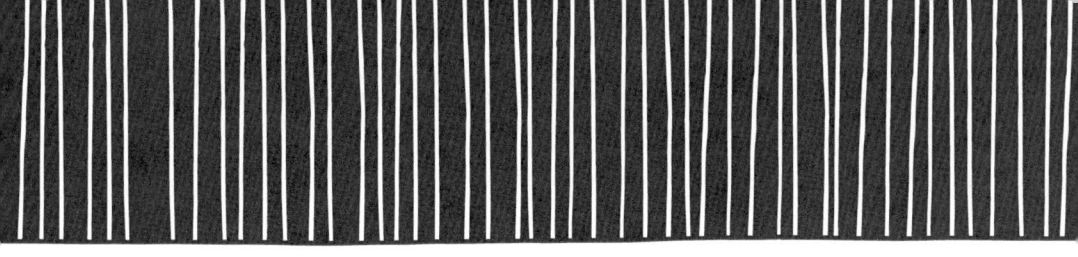

CHAPTER 4:

Mindless vs Mindful behavior

When one is paying attention and is in the present moment, that is an example of mindful behavior, however when one is absent from purpose, or is showing little or no attention that is an example of mindless behavior.

In order to combat mindless behavior, I recommend practicing these 4 techniques:

- Practice Gratitude
- Positive Affirmations
- Journaling
- Meditation

Learn what mindfulness is, work through the steps, and then discuss the opportunities and challenges you may face in your community.

I invite you to practice these techniques for four-weeks by incorporating each of these health practices on a weekly basis. All of these are interconnected and can impact your decision-making, even in things that may not seem health-related in any way. Here are a few recommendations:

Mindfulness/Gratitude/Affirmations/Journaling

What are the keys to your wellbeing?

Are you able to disconnect and recharge?

Here are a few topics to help you to discover your wellness by paying attention and being "IN" the moment.

Eating Mindfully (nutrition)

Dancing Mindlessly (physical)

Shopping Mindfully (meal plan prep)

Sleeping Mindfully (rest restore)

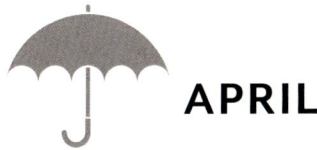 **APRIL**

April's is all learning to: Let go (lent) and the theme color is Teal Umbrellas.

April has several holiday/events such as April Fools Day, Earth day, & National Poetry month. My recommendation this month is to (Get out, & Garden)

This month is all about Assessments, so now it's time to reassess where you are in this journey since you've started from January. Celebrate your achievements and remember to keep it going and don't give up! I also recommend Practice giving up something for 30 days and replace that habit with a new one.

April's muscle of the month is the Gluteus Maximus, also known as the Glutes, located in the buttocks, or behind. Try doing Squats, and Donkey Kick Backs to strengthen and build up your Gluteus muscles.

Happy Birthday to everyone celebrating a birthday this month!

April Goal Sheet

I am mindful of my wellness and I plan today to be well today by doing the following things:

1.

2.

3.

Fill in the blank...

My wellness is:_____

My own responsibility: _____
My own right: _____
My own journey: _____

I empower _____

I educate _____

I help _____

I heal _____

I care _____

I am B-Wellness365 your name: _____

For this month, my goal is to _____

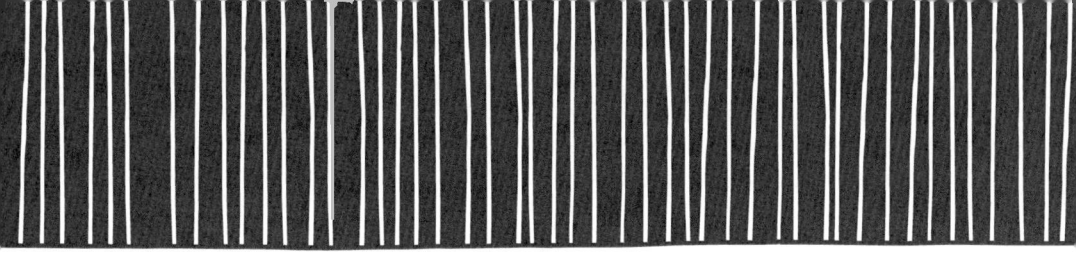

CHAPTER 5:

Stress overload

Time for a Transformation

In this chapter, we will learn how to transform from a caterpillar to a butterfly with a changed mindset. Which of these topics causes you to feel stress that you tend to focus on the most?

Community
Family
Acceptance
Personal connections with people
Uplifting
Coming together
Sharing stories
Non-judgments
Get grounded
Connecting broken pieces
Discuss
Intimacy
Sense of belonging
Strong teams
Feeling relief
Fellowship
Togetherness
Reshape our Thinking
Separate pieces to make whole
Life source
Joining forces

Making new friends
Negative Energy
Change
Opening up
Different perspectives

Circle the ones that resonate with you the most because these are the categories that need to be transformed from stressed, to stress-free.

Free yourself from these stressful overloads!

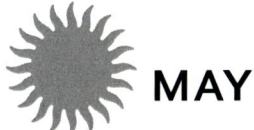 **MAY**

This month's theme is Mastery Movement May

May holidays/events include: Cinco de Mayo, Mother's Day, and Memorial Day.

May's color theme is a bright Yellow and the sun is this month's symbol.

I recommend eating vibrant yellow foods such as lemons, yellow bell peppers and squash.

Our theme this month in May is Mastery, so for this month try our Mindfulness/Movement/Memory 35 Exercise Poster Guide for 30 days and see if you can remember the techniques without using the pictures.

May's Muscle of the month is the Biceps, which are the muscles located in your arm. Try doing bicep curls with dumbbells or resistance bands.

Happy Birthday to everyone celebrating a birthday this month!

May Goal Sheet

I am mindful of my wellness and I plan today to be well today by doing the following things:

1.

2.

3.

Fill in the blank...

My wellness is:_____

My own responsibility: _____
My own right: _____
My own journey: _____

I empower _____

I educate _____

I help _____

I heal _____

I care _____

I am B-Wellness365 your name: _____

For this month, my goal is to _____

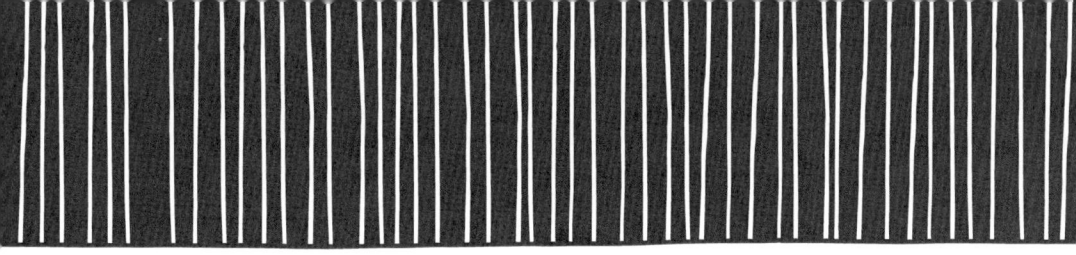

CHAPTER 6:

Meditation Minutes (M&M time to rest)

Making mindful decisions

Over 40 million people in the US suffer from anxiety and stress. Studies reveal that meditation helps reduce stress and improve quality of life.

Self-care has gained popularity and is being used as a preventive measure to help reduce stress levels.

Mindful practices can help individuals cope with stress and provide support for lifestyle changes that will help reduce stress.

Let's practice incorporating new attributes:

Mindful
Thoughtful
Thankful
Grateful
Graceful

What is your glass full of?

We can replace old habits and incorporate new ones. Remember it takes 21 days to create a habit and a lifetime of effort to maintain it!.

Let your commit to Wellness be a reminder everyday for your future. Continue to set your monthly goals and create lifestyle changes.

NOW IS THE TIME TO CONTINUE YOUR TRANSFORMATION!

I will be your accountability partner on this journey and will guide you with monthly tips and resources to help you achieve your goals!

Ready, Set, Lets Keep GOING!

Meditation

If meditation sounds intimidating, it's actually as simple as breathing. Join me to learn techniques on how the mind works, and even tap into this very process to find ways to relax and experience calmness. Currently research on meditation show that attention training can rewire the brain in ways that enhance cognition, emotion, performance, health and well being.

Meditation has a wide range of effects. It can help with focus, decreasing anxiety and stress, pain and boost immunity. It enhances cognitive function, like memory, concentration and mental stability, and mindful body awareness. It also decreases stress, and increases immune function and cortisol levels, which helps regulate energy levels, and much more.

How to Meditate (A beginner's step by step guide)

Practice this 4-week series of mindfulness topics everyday for self-awareness. Make the next 30 Days full of prosperity,

In this chapter you will:

- Learn meditation affirmations
- Take part in stretching and breathing exercises
- Learn movement and guided meditation exercises

Meditation helps you to:

Disconnect
Awareness
Breathe
Notice
Quieting the mind

Combine mindfulness meditation with short writing exercises for personal reflection I your journal and discover new our ways of being relaxed and let go and JUST BREATHE.

Here's how you meditate...

Sit comfortably with your back straight. Put one hand on your chest and the other on your stomach.

Breathe in through your nose. The hand on your stomach should rise.

The hand on your chest should move very little.

Exhale through your mouth, pushing out as much air as you can while contracting your abdominal muscles. The hand on your stomach should move in as you exhale, but your other hand should move very little.

Continue to breathe in through your nose and out through your mouth.

Try to inhale enough so that your lower abdomen rises and falls.

Count slowly as you exhale.

Guided sitting meditation, or a walking meditation (including walking outdoors, weather permitting) are equally effective as lying down

Learn ways to cultivate the power of stillness, power and strength through various standing and breathing techniques.

When things get hard, we have a tendency to want to run or to move, but true power lies deep within the stillness where the mind is clear and empty.

This activity is intended to guide you through simple but powerful techniques that will leave empowered and is great for people of all ages.

Learn ways to cultivate the power of stillness, power and strength through various standing and breathing techniques this month. Keep it going!

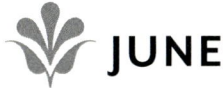 # JUNE

This month's theme is Joyful June

June has so much to celebrate! From graduations, to Fathers day, there's a lot to be joyful for this month. June's theme is all about Assessment time.

June's color theme is Lavender flowers. This month try using lavender, and eat purple foods like grapes, purple cabbage, and eggplant.

Since this is the halfway make for the program, you have been at this for 6 months now, let's check in to see how much progress you've achieved.

June's muscle of the month is the Gastronemus, which is located in the Calf.

Try doing Calf raises this month to strengthen and build up your calf muscles this month. It's a super easy exercise with no equipment necessary!

School's out and the kids are jumping for joy!

Happy Birthday to everyone celebrating a birthday this month!

June Goal Sheet

I am mindful of my wellness and I plan today to be well today by doing the following things:

1.

2.

3.

Fill in the blank...

My wellness is:_____

My own responsibility: _____
My own right: _____
My own journey: _____

I empower _____

I educate _____

I help _____

I heal _____

I care _____

I am B-Wellness365 your name: _____

For this month, my goal is to _____

PART 3

CHAPTER 7:

Choosing Wellness over wackiness

10 Effective Home Remedies For Water Retention

When our body feels out of balance, it could be that you are dehydrated, and need to drink water. If you feel out of whack, or off balance it could also be a sign of inflammation in the body.

Our bodies often retain water as a result of some internal issue in the body, and this condition is known as edema. Edema is most often manifested by swelling in the body.

Inflammation

If you're suffering from pain or swelling right now, take a hard look at what you're eating. Avoiding these inflammation-causing foods will have you feeling much better. Also, start incorporating some alkaline healthy foods into your diet and fruits/vegetables like blueberries, cherries, leafy greens, and tomatoes because they have the potential to reduce inflammation.

In order to eliminate water in the body, you should detect the cause of it, and take the needed steps to treat it, instead of just ignoring the symptoms.

Here are 12 ways to treat water retention: Try these recommendations:

1. Limit Sodium intake

2. Increase water intake

3. Sweat it off

4. Eat fruits, & veggies (natural diuretic)

5. Drink parsley tea

6. Drink apple cider vinegar

7. Drink Cranberry juice

8. Try Dandelions

9. Try Fennel Seeds

10. Epsom salt bath

11. Stinging Nettle root

12. Lemon juice

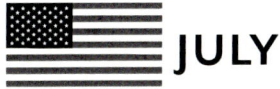 **JULY**

This month's theme is Just July

July's color theme is Red/White/ Blue Multiple colors flag, which signifies freedom and justice. It is all about Independence Day month & Parents day month (7/24)

July's muscle of the month is Abdominals so this month work on your abdominal muscles by doing crunches, sit-ups for your upper abs and reverse curls for the lower abs. This month try eating Plums, Berries (Blueberries, Blackberries) in your smoothies.

Happy Birthday to everyone celebrating a birthday this month!

July Goal Sheet

I am mindful of my wellness and I plan today to be well today by doing
the following things:

1.

2.

3.

Fill in the blank...

My wellness is:_____

My own responsibility: _____

My own right: _____

My own journey: _____

I empower _____

I educate _____

I help _____

I heal _____

I care _____

I am B-Wellness365 your name: _____

For this month, my goal is to _____

CHAPTER 8:

Just Breathe

Sometimes in the midst of our daily grind, it's possible to find ourselves holding our breath. Even more so, it can be hard to give yourselves permission to relax and let go of the increasing pressures and responsibilities of life. You must make a conscious effort to pay attention to your breath and be mindful of how you feel.

Mindful Breathing

Research shows that people who disconnect daily reported lower levels of stress and higher levels of well being.

What's your focus? Do you pay attention to yourself breathing?

Try listening to Guided Meditations For better sleep and mental clarity

Find a place to connect with people
A place to talk, meditate and share
A place to refresh, renew, readjust
Reset and rebalance your energy

<u>Set your intentions to improve your health</u>

Manage stress
Sleep better
Help with anxiety
Help improve energy levels

The Power of Paying Attention (POPA)

Mindfulness according to me....

Is to be in the moment (John Kabit Zinn

In the Zone (auto zone)

In the pocket (famous ball player)

Being totally engrossed in what you're doing at that exact time without distractions

Ignoring all things in order to stay focused on what you feel and what you're doing at that particular moment

Being on pointe

On ONE

Transformation happening in you

Learn to block out things/distractions/people

Retraining the brain

Mental Rest

Practice stillness

Working from a place of rest

Inner restoration

Recycling energy

Empty out the head load

Aware of mental state

Developing awareness

Blanking/ Blackout

Releasing Burdens

Inner rest

Administering Peaceful thoughts

Thought-Less Ness

Mindfulness is exercise for your mental/physical and spiritual health

Staying in rest

Living mentally free

Mental healing

Wisdom Wellness

Taking it to a whole other level of healing

Nothing can interrupt your ability to get clear from the inside out

Mindfulness is to Live from a place of rest

Focus on who you are, where you are and what you are currently doing

Mindfulness/Movement/ Memory Poster Guide

Mindfulness Movement & Memory Techniques for strength, balance, coordination and neurological improvement

Mindfulness Techniques
Focus and Attention

Movement Techniques
Chair Pilates and Cardiovascular Activities
To Keep The Body Active

Memory Techniques
Concentration and Neurological Behavior Management

Creating a system of health and self care processes for teaching wellness that is accessible and value driven which are evidence based.

Wellness sectors are no longer separate industries. They will increasingly converge as we integrate wellness into our homes and communities, our work, and our travel. All wellness sectors are dynamic and interconnected, intrinsically linked to the wellness economy.

Try these Mindfulness Movement & Memory Techniques everyday this month of July.

Mindfulness Holistic 12 Steps To B-Wellness365

Self-care & Stress Management Tips & Tools for healthy living

1. Affirmations
2. Breathing Techniques
3. Detoxification
4. Nutrition
5. Measurements
6. Meal Planning
7. Assessments
8. Physical Activity
9. Goal Setting
10. Accountability
11. Recipes for success
12. Meditation

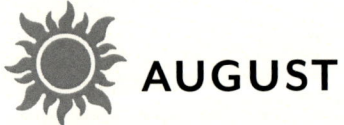

AUGUST

This month's theme is Awesome August

August theme is Fun in the sun and color theme is Tan neutral beige (sandy beaches)

August Muscle of the month is Triceps. Try doing Table tops, Dips, or Triceps extensions to target the back of your arm. August is friendship day (8/7), & national parks month, & national dog day 8/26.

This month try eating a peach or make a healthy shake with a peach.

Happy Birthday to everyone celebrating a birthday this month!

August Goal Sheet

I am mindful of my wellness and I plan today to be well today by doing the following things:

1.

2.

3.

Fill in the blank...

My wellness is:_____

My own responsibility: _____

My own right: _____

My own journey: _____

I empower _____

I educate _____

I help _____

I heal _____

I care _____

I am B-Wellness365 your name: _____

For this month, my goal is to _____

PART 4

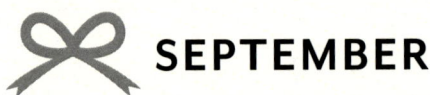 # SEPTEMBER

This month's theme is September's Scholars

September's theme is Back to basics. September's theme color is Pink, the symbol is ribbon and it's back to school season.

September muscle of the month is Hamstring, which is located in the back of the leg behind the knee. Try lying on your stomach and doing Leg Curls, or Toe Taps standing to target the hamstring muscles.

September is Childhood Obesity month, Labor Day, national grandparents day, 9/11, & patriots day/Remembrance Day/ Fall festivals.

This month also celebrates Fall Festivals and apple picking season.

I recommend trying a pink apple, grapefruit, watermelon or dragon fruit. They are all delicious!

Happy Birthday to everyone celebrating a birthday this month!

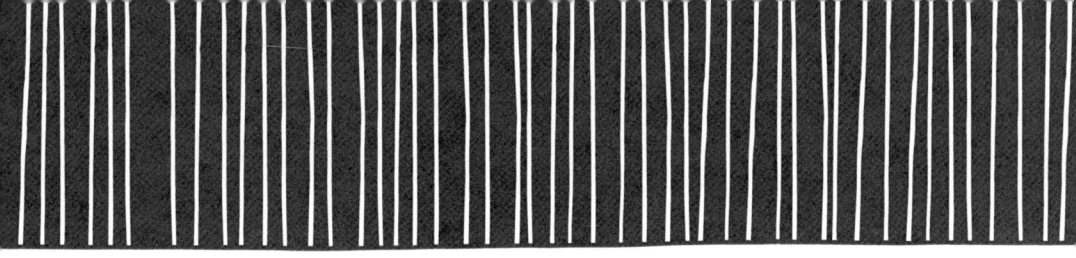

CHAPTER 9:

"What is Wellness?"

Wellness encompasses the biological, psychological, social, and spiritual aspects of person-in-environment functioning.

The origin of wellness: According to the World Health Organization, Wellness is defined as "the quality or state of being healthy in body and mind, especially as the result of deliberate effort.

OR

an approach to healthcare that emphasizes preventing illness and prolonging life, as opposed to emphasizing treating diseases.

Adverb
In a good or satisfactory manner:

thoroughly, carefully, or soundly:

Adjective, comparative better, superlative best.
In good health; sound in body and mind:

satisfactory, pleasing, or good:

Origin of Wellness
Before 900; Middle English, Old English well (l) (adj. and adv.); cognate with Dutch well, German wohl, Old Norse vel, Gothic waila

Synonyms for wellness

Well-being
Wholeness

Strength
Robust
Fitness
Vigor

September Goal Sheet

I am mindful of my wellness and I plan today to be well today by doing the following things:

1.

2.

3.

Fill in the blank...

My wellness is:_____

My own responsibility: _____
My own right: _____
My own journey: _____

I empower _____

I educate _____

I help _____

I heal _____

I care _____

I am B-Wellness365 your name: _____

For this month, my goal is to _____

CHAPTER 10:

Think about what you're thinking about

Grow Towards Wellness

This month continue to grow towards your wellness goals and commit to live a healthy and fulfilling life. Wellness is more than being free from illness: it is a process of change and growth towards a mentally and physically healthy lifestyle.

Your Health & Wellness Matters

In order to live a higher quality life, maintaining optimal wellness is key. Everything we feel and do relate to our well-being and directly affects our actions and emotions. In order to subdue stress, reduce illness, and ensure positive moments in your life, you must achieve optimal wellness.

Live With Passion & Purpose

To achieve optimal wellness, one must apply it towards every possible endeavor. You can apply a wellness approach towards your environment, community, career, belief systems, physical activities, self-care, healthy eating, self-esteem, and creative activities. Applying wellness in your everyday life will allow you to achieve your full potential and live with passion and purpose.

How do you plan on continuing to excess in your wellness journey?

Share your thoughts here: (Think about what you're thinking about)

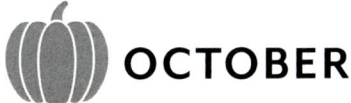 **OCTOBER**

This month's theme is Occasionally October.

October's theme color is Orange and symbol is a pumpkin

This month try eating bright foods such as carrots, orange bell pepper, pumpkin and oranges.

October has plenty of fun themed occasions, such as pumpkin picking season, apple picking, fall festivals and Halloween.

October muscle of the month is the quadriceps.

Try doing Lunges or Wall squats to target the front leg muscles.

October: Screenings

October Breast Cancer awareness month

Columbus Day, & Halloween

Happy Birthday to everyone celebrating a birthday this month!

October Goal Sheet

I am mindful of my wellness and I plan today to be well today by doing the following things:

1.

2.

3.

Fill in the blank...

My wellness is:_____

My own responsibility: _____
My own right: _____
My own journey: _____

I empower _____

I educate _____

I help _____

I heal _____

I care _____

I am B-Wellness365 your name: _____

For this month, my goal is to _____

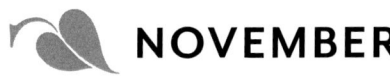 NOVEMBER

This month's theme is No Negativity November and Being thankful

November's muscle of the month is the Pectorals. Try doing pushups or dumbbell fly with weights to target the chest area.

November is Veterans Day & Thanksgiving, Election Day

November's color theme is Brown, Yellow, & Green leaves are the symbol

This month try eating wheat germ or flax seeds or Golden apples.

Happy Birthday to everyone celebrating a birthday this month!

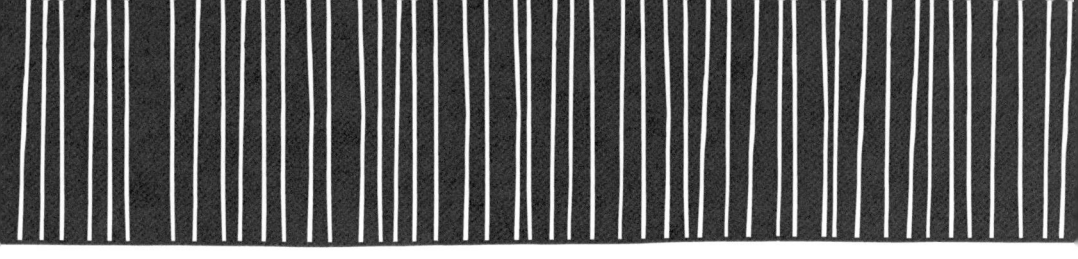

CHAPTER 11:

Ways to Stay Healthy

Monthly Challenges (3,7,14, &21 day)

Detox
Meditation
Push-up
Curl-up
Smoothie
Dips
Juicing

Meatless Monday's
Water (60ounces daily)
Language
Never Scared (Facing fears)
Gratitude (giving gifts of gratitude)
Hat (Women wear many hats)
Take a flick every day wearing different hats that represent your mood/job/vibe

The B-Wellness365 Monthly Health Challenges combines exercise classes with nutritional counseling and motivation into a well thought out system designed to help you dramatically improve your health, fitness, and appearance. This book is created for busy people. We have helped people achieve all sorts of different goals and we're here for you when you're ready!

1. Make the most crucial health information accessible to everyone with this simple health guidebook.

2. Each month of this health journal calendar is complete with tips for healthy living, wholesome nutrition and exercise fitness accompanied by full-color photography.

3. Ample space is provided for jotting notes, appointments and health reminders.

4. Perfect for keeping track of your wellness journey

Ways to Stay Healthy

What is Tai Chi

Gentle physical exercises done with rhythmic gentle flowing movements

Each posture flows into the next without pause, ensuring that your body is in constant motion. Tai chi has many different styles.

Taiji, short for Tai ji quan, or T'ai chi ch'üan, is an internal Chinese martial art practiced for both its defense training, its health benefits and meditation. The term taiji refers to a philosophy of the forces of yin and yang, related to the moves.

Tai chi: A gentle way to fight stress

Tai chi helps reduce stress and anxiety. And it also helps increase flexibility and balance.

If you're looking for a way to reduce stress, consider tai chi (TIE-CHEE). Originally developed for self-defense, tai chi has evolved into a graceful form of exercise that's now used for stress reduction and a variety of other health conditions. Often described as meditation in motion, tai chi promotes serenity through gentle, flowing movements.

What is tai chi?

Tai chi is an ancient Chinese tradition that, today, is practiced as a graceful form of exercise. It involves a series of movements performed in a slow, focused manner and accompanied by deep breathing.

Tai chi, also called tai chi chuan, is a non competitive, self-paced system of gentle physical exercise and stretching.

Each style may subtly emphasize various tai chi principles and methods.

There are variations within each style. Some styles may focus on health maintenance, while others focus on the martial arts aspect of tai chi.

Tai chi is different from yoga, another type of meditative movement. Yoga includes various physical postures and breathing techniques, along with meditation.

Who can do Tai Chi?

Tai chi is low impact and puts minimal stress on muscles and joints, making it generally safe for all ages and fitness levels. In fact, because tai chi is a low-impact exercise, it may be especially suitable if you're an older adult who otherwise may not exercise.

You may also find tai chi appealing because it's inexpensive and requires no special equipment. You can do tai chi anywhere, including indoors or outside. And you can do tai chi alone or in a group class.

Although tai chi is generally safe, women who are pregnant or people with joint problems, back pain, fractures, severe osteoporosis or a hernia should consult their health care provider before trying tai chi.

Modification or avoidance of certain postures may be recommended.

Why try tai chi?

When learned correctly and performed regularly, tai chi can be a positive part of an overall approach to improving your health. The benefits of tai chi may include:

- Decreased stress, anxiety and depression
- Improved mood
- Improved aerobic capacity
- Increased energy and stamina
- Improved flexibility, balance and agility
- Improved muscle strength and definition

More research is needed to determine the health benefits of tai chi. Some evidence indicates that tai chi may also help:

- Enhance quality of sleep
- Enhance the immune system
- Help lower blood pressure
- Improve joint pain
- Improve symptoms of congestive heart failure
- Improve overall well-being
- Reduce risk of falls in older adults

How to get started with tai chi

Although you can rent or buy videos and books about tai chi, consider seeking guidance from a qualified tai chi instructor to gain the full benefits and learn proper techniques.

You can find tai chi classes in many communities today. To find a class near you, contact local fitness centers, health clubs and senior centers.

A tai chi instructor can teach you specific positions and breathing techniques. An instructor can also teach you how to practice tai chi safely, especially if you have injuries, chronic conditions, or balance or coordination problems. Although tai chi is slow and gentle, and generally doesn't have negative side effects, it may be possible to get injured if you don't use the proper techniques.

After learning tai chi, you may eventually feel confident enough to do tai chi on your own. But if you enjoy the social aspects of a class, consider continuing with group tai chi classes.

Maintaining the benefits of tai chi

While you may gain some benefit from a tai chi class that lasts 12 weeks or less, you may enjoy greater benefits if you continue tai chi for the long term and become more skilled.

You may find it helpful to practice tai chi in the same place and at the same time every day to develop a routine. But if your schedule is erratic, do tai chi whenever you have a few minutes. You can even practice the soothing mind-body concepts of tai chi without performing the actual movements when you are in a stressful situation, such as a traffic jam or a tense situation.

November Goal Sheet

I am mindful of my wellness and I plan today to be well today by doing the following things:

1.

2.

3.

Fill in the blank...

My wellness is:_____

My own responsibility: _____
My own right: _____
My own journey: _____

I empower _____

I educate _____

I help _____

I heal _____

I care _____

I am B-Wellness365 your name: _____

For this month, my goal is to _____

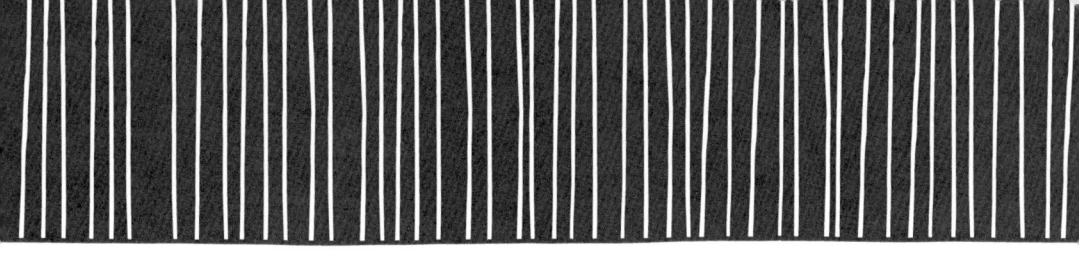

CHAPTER 12:

Herbs and Vitamins

Know your Vitamin foods

This month we discuss Herbs, and Vitamins.

Fruits and vegetables contain many vitamins and minerals that are good for your health. These include vitamins), C and E.

A: helps with vision (sweet potatoes
B: metabolism (Pistachios)
C: iron absorption (bell pepper)
D: helps immune system (salmon)
E: heart health (Sun flower seeds)
J: joy happiness, laughter
K: fights against blood clotting (good for circulation)

Vitamin A is a substance that the body needs in order to maintain proper health. It plays an important role in healthy vision, regulates genes, maintains healthy skin, and produces red blood cells, thus it supports the immune system and helps fight infections.

The body does not naturally produce vitamin A, which means that you need to make sure you are getting it from your diet. The recommended daily intake for men is 900 mcg, and for women, it's 700 mcg.

Vitamin A foods:

Broccoli,Carrots,Sweet Potato, Iceberg Lettuce,Salmon,Goat Cheese,Hard Boiled Egg,Mango, Mustard Greens, Butternut Squash, Kale, Grapefruit

Spices with vitamin A: Paprika, Dried Basil

Vitamin B is found in a variety of foods such as meat, wholegrains, and fruits. There are 8 vitamins — called B complex vitamins.

They are thiamine (B1), riboflavin (B2), niacin (B3), pantothenic acid (B5), pyridoxine (B6), biotin (B7), folate (B9) and cobalamin (B12).

They each have a unique function, and help your body produce energy and make important molecules in your cells.

A food must contain at least 20% of the Reference Daily Intake (RDI) per serving in order to be considered high in vitamin B

Vitamin B foods: Salmon, Greens, Liver, Eggs, Milk, Beef, Oysters, Clams, Mussels, Legumes, Chicken, Turkey, Yogurt, Sunflower Seeds

1. Whole grains (brown rice, barley, millet)
2. Meat (red meat, poultry, fish)
3. Eggs and dairy products (milk, cheese)
4. Legumes (beans, lentils) • Black beans
5. Chickpeas (garbanzo beans)
6. Edamame (green soybeans)
7. Green peas
8. Kidney beans
9. Lentils
10. Pinto beans
11. Roasted soy nuts

Vitamin B foods

Seeds and nuts (sunflower seeds, almonds)

Dark, leafy vegetables (broccoli, spinach, kale, turnip greens, lettuce, spinach, collard greens and lettuce

Fruits (citrus fruits, avocados, bananas)

B7 - barley, brewer's yeast, royal jelly, wheat bran, broccoli, cauliflower, legumes, mushrooms and spinach.

B9 -oranges, asparagus, bananas, melons, lemons, legumes, yeast, and mushrooms.

B12- bladderwrack, dandelion, alfalfa, and white oak bark.

Vitamin C foods:red bell peppers, broccoli, guava, oranges, lemon, orange juice, papaya, and strawberries.

Vitamin D, also known as the "sunshine vitamin," is widely known for its essential role in maintaining strong bones, yet there is so much more it does for our health.

Vitamin E is a powerful antioxidant that protects the skin, and hair against damage and is available as a supplement or oil. It also has been know to slow the aging process of cells, according to the National Institute of Health.

Vitamin K helps heal the body against wounds and helps in certain skin conditions such as stretch marks, spider veins, and bruises which is great for circulation and blood flow.

HERBS for Detoxing

Many herbs can be used to stimulate and cleanse your uterus, improve its tone and ease menstrual or menopausal symptoms.

Every single ingredient has scientifically-proven properties to ease symptoms: naturally. Here are a few recommendations.

Ashwagandha has been found to inhibit the formation of beta-amyloid plaques in preliminary research.

Bladderwort has been used to treat fluid retention, urinary tract disorders, and kidney stones.

Dandelion Root: reduced fasting blood glucose levels by 29.9% in a 2016 clinical study

Elderberry is good for cold and flu. It reduces inflammation and strengthens the immune System. This is a commonly taken remedy in traditional Chinese medicine (TCM)

Fennel Seed is know as "mother nature's secret weapon" for supporting healthy blood sugar.

Ginger is a whole-body detoxifier because it supports liver function, boosts circulation and promotes healthy sweating. Ginger also has been known to lower blood glucose levels by 17%, LDL levels by 12%[2] in a major study of diabetic patients and reduces inflammation while increasing oxygen and blood flow.

Lavender Petals: relaxes, helps with sleep, keeps high blood sugar in check

Marigold is a good cleansing herb that can be used to support uterine health

Drinking marigold tea, or combining marigold and chamomile in tea, can help regulate menstrual bleeding and ease cramps.

Motherwort has been used in used in traditional Chinese medicine to treat menopausal and menstrual symptoms and may help the uterus contract after giving birth.

Sage may possess memory-enhancing properties, and may aid in the treatment of Alzheimer's disease. Try adding sage to butternut squash, roasted chicken, turkey, tomato sauce, or in a white bean soup. Sage can also be consumed in tea form.

Sencha reduces blood glucose levels in the digestive tract

Stevia Leaf: the only all-natural sweetener that's not harmful to diabetics also supports healthy blood sugar and increases insulin resistance.

Turmeric is a spice long used in Ayurveda. It contains a compound called curcumin, which has antioxidant and anti-inflammatory effects (two factors that may benefit brain health and overall health). Turmeric is a key ingredient in curry powder, which typically also includes such spices as coriander and cumin. To increase your intake of turmeric, try adding curry powder or turmeric to stir-fries, soups, and vegetable dishes. Turmeric Root has been linked in over 190 studies to maintaining healthy blood sugar levels and supporting healthy insulin function

Tulsi: supports insulin levels and reduces glucose levels in the body.

This month try one or more of these Herbs and share your opinion on how they make you feel.

My advise for a healthy life

Eliminate mucus & toxins from your body

Laugh often

Drink 1/2 your body weight in ounces of water daily

Surround yourself with positive people

Exercise, Dance or be physically active

Drink, Eat fruits and vegetables

Detox monthly

Read, Rest and Reset

Bonus advise... smile often

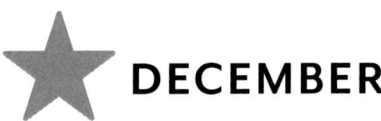 # DECEMBER

This month's theme is Definitely Delicious December

December's theme is Family first. This month is muscle is the Trapezius muscle, also known as the Christmas tree muscle because of its shape and location on the back. Try bent over rows or cobra position to target the trapezius muscles.

December is also Hanukkah, Kwanzaa, Christmas, & New Years Eve month

December's color theme is Platinum tree decorated with gold wreath, & a gold star.

Since this month is definitely delicious, I recommend that you indulge in the most tastiest foods (in moderation of course) however, swapping sweets can be helpful this month. Try using brown sugar instead of white, also replace artificial sweeteners with banana, natural honey, agave or dates when baking.

Adding dry fruit is very popular this month like apricots, raisins and cranberries to desserts.

Happy Birthday to everyone celebrating a birthday this month!

December Goal Sheet

I am mindful of my wellness and I plan today to be well today by doing the following things:

1.

2.

3.

Fill in the blank...

My wellness is:_____

My own responsibility: _____

My own right: _____

My own journey: _____

I empower _____

I educate _____

I help _____

I heal _____

I care _____

I am B-Wellness365 your name: _____

For this month, my goal is to _____

Eating Mindfully (Mind-Body Nutrition Program

(Eating & Physical Activity)

Here are recommendations for beginning a detox.

1st 7days are no chewing days
Day 1-3 detoxification, blood cleanse, remove toxins from the body
Day 4-7 incorporates juices, smoothies, tea, & soup
Day 8-15 meal prepping, incorporate lean proteins and vegetables
Day 16-21 incorporating carbohydrates and healthy fats

Approved foods for 21 day Cleanse eating
Water consumption must be 1/2 your body weight in ounces.
Start with 20 ounces of water, day 1-3 then gradually increase by day 4-7 double the water intake to 40 ounces

By day 8, you should be drinking 50ounces

Watermelon
Cucumber
Tomatoes
Cantaloupe
Celery
All Berries (strawberries, blueberries, raspberries, blackberries)
Cherry
Apple
Peaches
Oranges
Clementines
Grapefruit
Pomegranate
Pear
Plum
Grapes

Avocado
Juneberries (June plum)
1/2 a banana per day (Blue Java Bananas)

Non-Vegetarians Food Menu Options

Fish 3X per week minimum
Chicken 1-2X per week
Eggs
Tuna, Shrimp, Cod, Salmon
Beef or Pork (1 day per week)
1 Day of Vegetarian (no meat, fish) ex. Meatless Monday

Beans (garbanzo, red, black, green, pinto, Butter, Lima)
Bell Peppers (red,yellow,green)
Cabbage
Zucchini
Squash
Pumpkin
Sweet Potato
Potatoes
Carrots
Beets
Quinoa
Soups
Oatmeal
Peanut or Almond butter
Crackers
Green Leafy vegetables
Spinach
Kale
Brussel Sprouts
Collard greens
Broccoli
Green Beans
Water Cresses
Arugula
Turnip Greens
Swiss Chard

Dandelion Greens
Mustard Greens
Cállaloo
Lettuce
Leeks

Eating Mindfully

Breakfast/Lunch/Dinner/Snack Recommendations

7 Breakfast choices

Eggs, Toast,Avocado
Oatmeal,raisins,apple slices,cinnamon,nutmeg
Cereal (Bran flakes,Milk of Choice)
Almond, Coconut, Soy,Rice,Non-Dairy
Whole wheat pancakes with fruit
Smoothie
Home fries (Potatoes, Omelette, peppers/onion)

7 Lunchtime choices

Tuna on Rye,Wheat
Salad with Protein & Vinaigrette
Hummus With crackers, carrots, Bell peppers
Variety of soups
Lentil/Tomate/Chicken Noodle/Carrot Ginger/ Miso/ Beet/Green Pea

7 Dinnertime choices

Jerk Salmon with brown rice,& cabbage
Baked Potatoes with Roasted vegetables and (non vegetarian may add protein)
Soup
Zucchini pasta
Eggplant Parmigiana w/Roasted Vegas
Garlic Shrimp & Broccoli
Tofu fried rice with/ or with out protein
Chickpea salad w/peppers &almond slices

7 Snack choices

Cinnamon Almonds/Pistachios/Walnuts/No salt peanuts
Cran Raisins/ or golden raisins

Cereal

Fruit Smoothie
Carrot with Celery with peanut butter or hummus
2 Oatmeal raisin cookies

Banana Bread
Corn bread with corn & red peppers
Carrot Loaf with walnuts
Coconut Lime Loaf
Lemon Loaf
Dark chocolate Loaf

Shopping Mindfully

Approved Liquids

Water
Coconut water
Green tea
Iced tea
Lemonade
Smoothies
Cranberry juice
Non dairy milk (coconut/almond/rice/soy)
Orange Grapefruit Juice
Carrot Juice
Sorrel
Teas (peppermint/lemon/matcha/chai/black)

Spices

Turmeric
Garlic
Basil
Onions
Curry
Cinnamon
Nutmeg
Pepper flakes
Lemons
Limes
Apple cider vinegar
Olive oil
Dijon Mustard

Meal Plan & Prep

Try to Limit or minimize these items:

Dairy
Artificial sweets
Carbonated drinks
Caffeine
Sodium (salt)
Sugar
Minimum alcohol. No more than 2glasses per week

Banana only allowed 1/2 in a smoothie or in cereal
Replace sugar with these items instead:
Agave,Honey

Brown sugar is ok in moderation, organic coconut sugar, guava

Eat Alkaline Foods that contain water because it helps keep the body hydrated. Try the following items:

Tomatoes
Cucumber
Watermelon
Pineapple
Cantaloupe

Meal Planning and Prepping can help you organize your meals beforehand and saves you time, money and reduces food waste.

Are you open to sticking to a meal plan? Share your thoughts.....

Shopping Mindfully

More Tips & Tricks

Buy quality, delicious natural and organic products. No artificial flavors, colors, preservatives, sweeteners or hydrogenated fats will ever be in any of the food we sell. Meat will still come from animals raised with no-added growth hormones, ever. And all eggs in our dairy cases will continue to come from cage-free hens that aren't given antibiotics.

Kale Recipe

Kale is an excellent green to use in your healthy fruit smoothie recipes. Kale is related to cabbage, broccoli and Brussels sprouts and has a flavor that is more suggestive of broccoli.

Nutrition and Health Benefits

Kale contains beta-carotene, vitamin K, vitamin C, lutein, calcium and fiber. A sulfur-containing phytonutrient in kale called sulforaphane is believed to have powerful anti-cancer, anti-diabetic and anti-microbial properties and is released when the leaves are chopped or chewed (or blended in a green smoothie!) Kale also contains powerful antioxidants that help protect against certain cancers such as ovarian cancer. Kale is an excellent green to use for detox smoothies as it has cleansing properties. The nutrients in kale help protect against cataracts while promoting healthy lungs, cardiovascular health and boosts the immune system. Kale has anti-inflammatory properties making it an excellent food for those with rheumatoid arthritis.

How To Select Kale

Choose kale with deeply colored green leaves that are firm and do not show signs of wilting, yellowing or browning. Kale is available all year.

Using Kale In Green Smoothies

Kale has a slightly stronger flavor than baby spinach, so if you are not used to green smoothies, you might want to use strongly flavored fruit such as strawberries or pineapple to help mask the flavor. You can also slowly introduce kale into your smoothie recipes and increase the amount to two cups per recipe over time. I enjoy the flavor of kale in my green smoothies. Kale has a firmer texture than spinach as well, so you might need to blend your shake slightly longer if you are not using a high-end Vita-Mix blender.

Kale Smoothie Recipes

Here are some great kale green smoothie recipes I recommend:

Kale, coconut, orange strawberries.1 cup cleaned, pealed if necessary.

Blend until rich and smooth. This smoothie recipe contains over 30% of your daily value of calcium and is a great complement to a healthy breakfast.

Here are a few other kale recipes to try.

Kale, Orange & Strawberry Smoothie
Kale, Pineapple & Mint Smoothie
Kale, Mango, & Avocado Smoothie
Kale, Apple, & Carrot Smoothie
Kale, Peach, & Pear Smoothie
Kale, Bananas , & Spinach Smoothie
Kale, Lemon & Honey Smoothie

Enjoy Kale-ing!

Brownie Wellness Fruit Pizza Recipe

This healthy Brownie Fruit Pizza taste like real brownies: a delicious fudgy chocolate brownie pizza crust loaded with creamy coconut yogurt, coconut shreds and fruits. It is an allergy friendly dessert, 100% Paleo, eggs free, dairy free and grain free.

BROWNIE WELLNESS FRUIT PIZZA: PALEO, VEGAN AND GLUTEN FREE

Here's a quick and easy healthy treat for low carb and gluten free brownies lovers.

If you love chocolate for dessert then you must try this low carb Fudgy Avocado Brownie because they are sugar-free, delicious fudgy chocolaty flavor and crunchy walnuts. You'll love that those avocado brownies are a one-bowl blender recipe ready in few minutes.

I enjoy using avocado in my recipes because it provides an incredible fudgy texture to brownies, with no aftertaste at all. You must use a very ripe avocado to avoid lumps and obtain the right texture. If your avocado doesn't ripe very well store them near bananas at room temperature for few days in a brown bag.

My gift to you..... with Love..... "Brownie Wellness"

Essential Oils 12 month recommendations

Sleeping Mindfully (Rest & Restore)

This month try incorporating essential oils for rest and relaxation. Here are 12 recommendations and it's health benefits.

Lavender: helpful for relaxing and soothing
Peppermint: good for head aches
Lemon grass: relieves pain and swelling
Eucalyptus: soothes physical discomforts, and is anti-inflammatory
Sandlewood: reduces blood pressure levels, creates relaxation and peace
Frankensense: reduces joint inflammation
Baby powder: soothing properties, calming effects
Orange Blossom: natural astringent. Simulates skin healing
Coconut: heals wounds, reduces acne
Cinnamon Spice: great for circulation and blood flow
Ocean: fresh, peaceful clean scent
Cherry: sweet aromatic and calming scent relaxes the body

Exercises 24 Movement Sequence

Name & description of Exercises:

Seated Pretzel
Sleeping Snail (childs pose)

Cobra (upward dog)
Downward Dog
3 Legged dog

Mountain
Sun Salutation

Forward fold
Prayer

Right arm extended
Left arm extended
Both arms extended

Tree (right/Left leg)
Chair Pose

1/2 Moon R
1/2 Moon L

Triangle (R)
Triangle (L)

Climb ropes
Prayer hands heart Head, sky, circle
Seated meditation

5 check points:
Feet
Knees
Hips
Shoulder
Head

Mindfulness meditation mantra

Peace is in me
Breathing balloon
Eyes closed

You have to awaken Peace,
You must acknowledge Peace
You must awaken Peace,
You must embrace Peace, nourish peace and most importantly, PROTECT Peace!

You have the ability to tap into your inner peace and activate it within yourself!

Repeat this meditation mantra several times if you need to protect your peace!

Share your thoughts of your experience.

Resources

This book is not just a health planner!

B-Wellness365 offers monthly tools that can help:
Track healthy habits
Create a priority focus
Develop a growth mindset
Develop Focus
Defeat Distraction
Daily Affirmations
Attitude of Gratitude
Flexible
Habit and Discipline Tracking

- Develop daily healthy habits with the weekly tracker
- Six basic disciplines with room to add more
- Grow at your own pace as you become more effective and efficient

Affirmations

- 80% or more of the average person's thoughts can be negative
- Train your brain toward opportunity, positivity, and growth.
- Space for 12 personalized affirmations

Goal Planning

- Identify how you will move toward your ideal goals
- Plan your personal, professional, health, and relationship goals for the next 3months.

- Identify key weekly milestones that will move you toward your goals
- Each week, rate your progress and identify ways to improve your results

Daily Focus

- Identify the daily priorities that will move you forward
- Mindset exercises to practice appreciation and positivity
- Identify potential distractions to grow your awareness of what erodes your time and energy.
- The daily ritual that will keep you focused on your goals and your mindset fixed on positivity and growth.

Night Review

- The most successful people in the world journal their thoughts daily
- Get your thoughts on paper about what went right, what went wrong, and how you can improve tomorrow.
- Keep a record of your progress and the story of your defined life.

Understand how food works together with your body to improve quality of life

Getting connected to like-minded people
Sharing life stories
Transformation
Redevelopment
Working progress

Health, Fitness & Dieting/Personal Health/Longevity

Health, Fitness & Dieting/Counseling & Psychology/Movements/
Cognitive Behavioral Therapy
Cognitive behavioral therapy
Health, Fitness & Dieting/Counseling & Psychology/Group Therapy

Family wellness initiative

B-Wellness365 Initiative is to provide families in underserved communities with training in how to teach parents and students in grades 2-12 to take care of their wellness with a wholesome holistic approach

This book provides step-by-step instruction that will help you implement a wellness measurement program that identifies your most successful recipes, maps your exercise journey, uncovers insights with in-depth health and nutrition guide.

My organization's theory of change aims to spread this global wellness program by teaching families outside formal evaluation systems

Education policy making

Linking health achievement to life outcomes

Show value-added

Impact students future outcomes

Health is the foundation for all

Focus on empowering families to learn and implement wellness strategies for themselves and their children

Youth Family & Health services

We are your 1 stop shop for family health education & empowerment

What's your families Health Plan?

What's your plan to stay healthy?

Incorporate these techniques for a stress free healthy lifestyle

Mindfulness
Yoga
Exercise
Walking
Gardening
Laughter
Sleep
Rest & Relaxation
Fellowship
Nutritious meals
Family
Community

Types of Classes

Check out our Weekly Classes at B-Wellness365

Mindful Monday's (Meditation) meatless
Turn up Tuesdays (Zumba)
Workshop Wednesday's (Weekly topics)
Tone&Tighten Thursday's
FriYAAy Friends (Bootcamp)
Soca Saturday's (Soca-fit)
Sun Salutations Sunday's (Yoga) seafood

We offer many classes so join us for our trial class. Some of our classes include:
Heart health (Cardiovascular
Muscles Strengthening
Flexibility (Lengthening)

Joint health (Anti inflammatory)
Oral health (dental hygiene)
Digestive health (Enzymes/Gut)
Brain Health (Memory)

Epidermis Health (Skin)
Hair Care (Healthy Hair Follicles)
Nail Health
Eye Health (Vision/ Corneas)
Lifestyle (sleep/diet/habits)
What to eat/ How to shop
Weight
Blood pressure
Cholesterol
Waist Circumference
Sleep
Stress
Assessments

About Ivette Brown

Hi, my name is Ivette Brown aka Brownie Wellness, founder of Wellness 365 nonprofit organization and creator of BBBWI Health and Wholeness Curriculum Guide.

I am a doctoral candidate, educator/entrepreneur, and Yoga Therapist that loves helping people. Health & Fitness is my life and I enjoy inspiring others to reach their goals. I also am a 25 year veteran in the health and fitness industry and have worked with many organizations, schools, religious organizations, on health/physical education providing my professional subject matter expertise. Currently I am pursuing a Doctorate Degree in K-12 Education & Administration at Seton Hall University in addition to running a non-profit and BBBWI while finishing up this book: BWellness365 Method: Health Planner. The anatomy of lifestyle.

Mind-Body approach to achieving holistic health

I've been inspired to write this book because I believe that young people are our future leaders and they should have access to mentorship, health and educational opportunities outside of school.

My goal is to motivate and inspire individuals to do something productive for themselves everyday for the rest of their lives. This personal commitment requires activating self awareness, personal development, patience and accountability. I have an amazing team of Wellness professionals that help me make communities healthy through several fitness classes, nutrition workshops, dance residences and employee wellness programs daily.

My organization also serve adult medical centers, active older adult senior centers ages 55&up, PreK-12 grade schools and students with special needs in Surrounding areas of NY, NJ from everyone ages of 7-97.

It is the hope that through BBBWI Enrichment offerings our students' imaginations, interests, knowledge, and love of learning will grow. Students will learn social skills, accountability and mindful nutrition and fitness training throughout the classes.

Join the Movement & Stay connected with Brownie Wellness

BWellness365 Wellness Initiative "Join the movement!"

This self care wellness program is for individuals or families to implement into their own lifestyle and teach to their children.

The purpose of this book is to provide health educational support to youth and families. My B-Wellness365 Initiative aims to provide families, education, training in nutrition/mindfulness and fitness so that they can learn how to take care of their wellbeing to prevent early onset diabetes, high blood pressure, high cholesterol, and obesity.

Check out our website
www.browniewellness.com

Follow us on Instagram
Browniewellness

Follow us on Facebook
Bodies By Brownie

Follow us on Twitter
@browniewellness

Subscribe to our YouTube channel
IveBrown

Subscribe to our newsletter

Subscribe to our blog
Ivette Brown

Bodies By Brownie Wellness Institute
www.browniewellness.com
347-675-4200

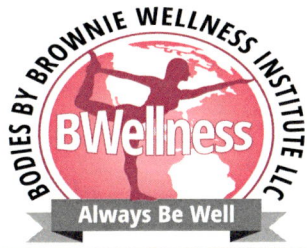

B-Wellness 365 Health Assessment

Name:_____Birthday:_____

Address_____ Age:_____

Email Address:_____

Phone #:_____ Relationship status:_____

Height:_____Weight:_____ Body Measurements:_____

Occupation:_____Children:_____ Pets:_____

Health Concerns:_____

Personal Wellness Goals:_____

Past Injuries/Illness/hospitalizations:_____

Ancestry:_____When did you feel your best:_____

How many hours do you sleep?_____Do you wake up at night?_____

Do you take Supplements?_____ Vitamins:_____Medications:_____

Do you suffer from allergies?_____How many meals do you eat daily?_____

Do you exercise?_____ If yes, what activities do you perform?_____

How often do you exercise?_____Do you have any cravings?_____

Bodies By Brownie Wellness Institute LLC
www.browniewellness.com
Phone: 347-675-4200 E-Mail: Ivette@browniewellness.com
Twitter: @browniewellness
Instagram: Browniewellness

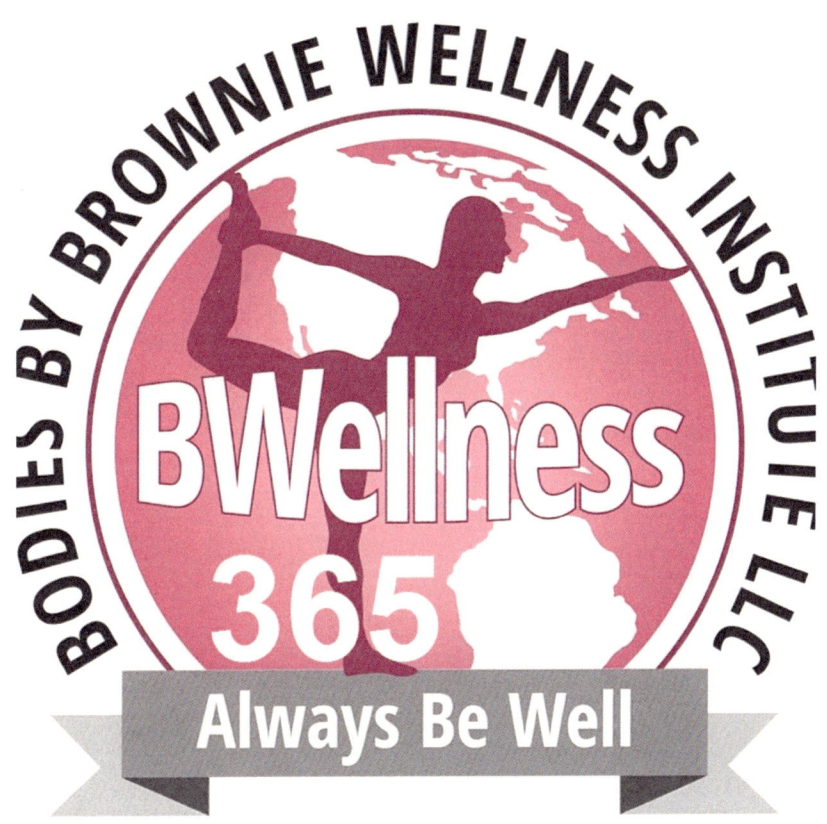

BODIES BY BROWNIE WELLNESS INSTITUE LLC

BWellness 365

Always Be Well